The Best Guide To Natural Hair

How To Begin Your Natural Hair Journey Today

Argena Hall

www.naturalhairmaster.com

Natural Hair Checklist & Journal [FREE]

Our printable checklist provides you with a list of everything you'll need to begin your natural hair journey.

Take it with you on the go, it can be downloaded on any device.

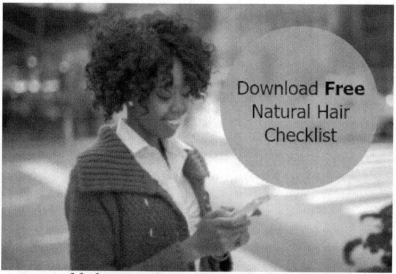

Download **Free** Natural Hair Checklist

As an added **BONUS** you'll receive our **Natural Hair Journey Journal**. A digital journal where you can track your experiences of growth, recipes, and more.

To Download Visit:
www.naturalhairmaster.com/naturalhaircheckli standjournal

Table of Contents

Introduction

I want to thank you and congratulate you for downloading the book, *"The Beginners Guide To Natural Hair: How To Begin Your Natural Hair Journey Today"*.

This book contains the exact information you need to start your natural hair journey.

It also includes the best ways to style your hair when you're first starting off (pictures included).

When I first started my journey, my hair was very thin and brittle and I was having a lot of breakage.

So I watched some natural hair videos on YouTube and pieced everything together.

Over the years, I've taken all I've learned and made my own routine to grow and care for my hair.

It's been a long time coming (about 3 years), but I've learned so much about how to grow and maintain my natural hair.

I put together this comprehensive guide on how to take care of your hair when you're just starting out because I know what it's like to start and not know what to do.

In this book, I go into how to maintain your hair so

it grows long over time.

Also, how to grow your hair natural without doing the "big chop."

There are tips on how to keep your hair healthy; and what things to avoid.

I also go into how to create a schedule of when you should do your hair. This is important because it will keep you on track so you don't neglect your hair.

We will also go into routines to follow before styling; such as hot oil treatments and deep conditioning.

Thanks again for downloading this book; you are now on your way to natural hair!

Why I Wrote This Book

I wrote this book because I remember what it's like to be lost and not know what the next step to take is. We are in the middle of a "natural revolution" where it's now praised to be natural and wear our hair curly, kinky, and coily.

Since there's a natural revolution going on, I knew that women like you would need a place to start.

After you decide you want to go natural; you then have to decide what to do next. What to do and what not to do. The best practices and treatments, etc.

To keep you from going crazy like I was, I decided to write a guide to help you start your natural journey off in a way that best suits you, your needs, and your schedule.

We all know that relaxers make your hair easier to manage and super straight. But we also know that they have harmful chemicals that can damage your hair drastically.

I wrote this book for the women who want to get started on their journey and never look back. Those women who look forward to loving their hair, treating it right and letting it be as kinky and or curly as it wants.

Chapter 1: Products You Need

Before starting your natural hair journey, there are going to be certain products you need in order to maintain your hair.

Also, because you're going natural; there are also some products you can now get rid of.

Keep in mind that some of these products may work for you, and some may not. It's up to you to **try and see what works best for your hair type.**

Upon trying different products, you'll find what works best for you. And who knows? You may hit a gold mine as far as what products treats your hair the way you want it.

You only want natural products that don't contain sulfate and other harmful chemicals that can strip your hair.

Going natural means using natural products... for the most part. But some products that aren't completely natural may be of benefit to your hair too. It depends on your hair type and what your hair responds best to.

No product is perfect, but after tons of research on the best products that will allow my hair to grow and keep it moisturized, I came up with a list.

You can also get a complete printable checklist by going to

http://www.naturalhairmaster.com/freechecklist

To start off, you're going to need only the basic products. I recommend that you start off with a simple hair style such as twists or a small curly fro. A small fro is also known as "teeny weeny afro or twa" in the natural world.

The first thing you're going to need is a conditioner. The conditioner is a must; invest in both a leave in conditioner and a wash out conditioner or a conditioner that is both.

Conditioners are important because it's what keeps your hair moisturized so it doesn't dry out.

Dry hair is the worst because it's causes breakage.

Conditioners

The best conditioners are Burts Bees, Herbal Essences and Olive Oil (in my opinion). They're all sulfate free.

Burts Bees

I tried Burt's Bees because I wanted to use something with more natural ingredients in it. I found that it's amazing!

When I do my deep conditions, it keeps my hair very soft and fluffy. Love it to death!

I think Burt's Bees is a best-kept secret for natural sistas! People of all races use it and I think the results are outstanding.

Herbal Essences

Herbal essences is a great conditioner too, I started off using it. It's more affordable and you can find coupons and everything for it.

I still buy Herbal Essences when it's on sale. And it smells amazing! I use the Hello Hydration conditioner and shampoo when buying Herbal Essences.

It does the job, but the conditioner doesn't work as well as others when I do my deep condition; as far as softening and detangling my hair and making it more manageable.

Olive Oil

The last one I use is Olive Oil, the kind you can wash out, and the kind you can put on dry hair and leave in.

We'll get more into styling later, but if you're going to use twists as one of your hairstyles, it's nice to have olive oil conditioner to use in your hair before styling.

Olive oil is, of course, a natural product and is pretty much safe for your hair in any form. So you can never go wrong with olive oil!

Shampoos

I hardly ever use shampoo anymore because I usually do a co-wash. A co-wash is when you replace a conditioner for your shampoo. The only time you really will need a shampoo is when you really need to clean your hair from product build up or dirt.

Of course, this varies depending on hair type. If you have oilier hair, then you should definitely shampoo a lot more than someone with more thick and dry hair.

When I do shampoo, I use are pretty much the same for the conditioners, except I haven't tried olive oil as a shampoo because it's not a cleanser, it's a moisturizer.

So I use Burts Bees and Herbal Essences.

They both get your hair clean. I don't think one is better than the other.

But I know Burt's Bees has more natural ingredients.

So if I had to go with one I would definitely choose Burt's Bees.

Deep Conditioner

You're going to want to pick up a deep conditioner for when you do your deep conditions.

The one I use is called Shea Moisture: Raw Shea Butter Restorative Conditioner. It contains sea kelp and argan oil.

Shea Moisture has a pretty decent line for black women. I recently started trying their products and I have realized more moisture in my hair.

The thing I like about this deep conditioner is that it's both a leave in a washout. Two products in one!

Deep conditioners will keep your hair from drying out and it helps repair any breakage.

Twisting Creams

As I mentioned earlier the best styles to start off with are twists or a curly fro; if at all applicable.

Unless your hair is super magic and will stay in twists by itself, you're going to need a twisting cream.

Some women have reported that they don't need a twisting cream, but I tried this and for my hair type-- the twists didn't last very long.

I've experimented with my share of twisting creams and my two favorites are Shea Moisture: Curl Enhancing Smoothie and Murray's Beeswax.

They're both pretty good but my favorite and the one I'm currently using is the Curl Enhancing Smoothie.

My hair has changed texture over the years, and I noticed the Organic Root Stimulator product that I used to use was starting to leave flaky residue in my hair.

But when I first started off, it was great. So what I'm thinking is the thicker and nappier your hair, the better the organic root stimulator will work.

And as you start deep conditioning and taking care of your hair you may find you need to change your twisting cream.

It's nice to experiment with what works best for you at the time.

So I say get them both and see which works best for you.

Hair Recipes

If you're the do it yourself type and really don't like to use store bought products, consider picking up my book Natural Hair Recipes. You can create your own natural hair products using simple natural ingredients.

Check it out here:

http://www.amazon.com/Natural-Hair-Recipes-Yourself-Products-ebook/dp/B00SNU3F8S/

Hair Accessories

To start off, you're going to need simple things like hair ties and lots and lots of headbands.

Headbands are great for the gym, for fashion, and they are a natural sista's dream!

I like to buy the thicker kind for when I'm wearing my fros, and the thinner kind for things like fashion and the gym.

They tend to stretch out after a while, so you'll find yourself replenishing them all the time.

You will also need shower caps, and a comb set with different sized combs for different styles. The one you'll use the most is a wide-tooth comb for detangling and a rat tooth comb for parting.

And for sleeping and styling reasons, you'll need a full-sized satin/silk scarf and a bonnet. Also, consider getting a satin pillowcase for those times you don't feel like wrapping up your hair at night.

The Take Away

These are the basic products you need to get started on your natural hair journey. If you truly want your hair to grow and be healthy use the recommended products or, at least, something similar that you know will work for you.

Chapter 2: Styling Your Hair

There are so many ways to wear your natural hair! The choices are infinite. Here are some of my favorite styles and instructions on how to do them.

I actually have a natural hair styles book in the making. Click here if you're interested in being featured.

If you're a visual learner I suggest you go to http://www.naturalhairmaster.com/ for step by step video tutorials.

Twists

Twists are by far the easiest, most stylish, and save you the most time. Depending on how small you make your twists they can last up to 2 weeks.

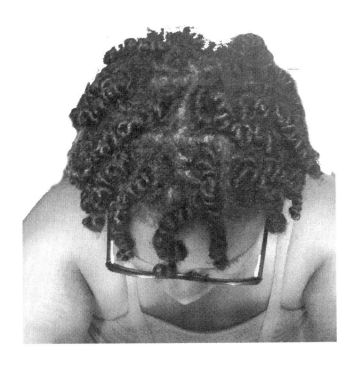

Keep in mind that twists are the way I grew my hair out. They allow your hair to breathe and are super easy to do once you get the hang of it.

Protective styles like twists and braids are great for growing out your hair. If you're looking for something low maintenance, try them out.

You can do it yourself or go to the shop.

For my size head (which is really big); it takes about an hour and a half to do them and I do medium sized twists.

How To Do Twists

First, make sure your hair is clean and moisturized, do a deep condition before you start your twists.

We will go into how to do a deep condition in Chapter 3.

You can do twists on dry hair or wet hair. The only difference I've found is wet hair lasts a bit longer and dry hair gives you more length.

Step #1: Take a small section of your hair (big enough to do one twist) and put some leave in conditioner through it, from top to bottom, so that the whole section gets conditioned. Then add some twisting cream to the tip of your fingers and apply it to the section.

Step #2: Separate the section into two even strands.

Step #3: Begin twisting the strand. Make sure when you're at the top you're doing your twists as close to your scalp as possible.

Make your twist as tight as possible.

Step #4: Once you get to the end of the strand, twist the end around your finger so that it won't come loose.

Then repeat this process until your whole head is finished.

Twist Out

The great thing about natural hair is how low maintenance it can be. After you leave your twists in for a week or two; you can then go straight into a twist out for another few days.

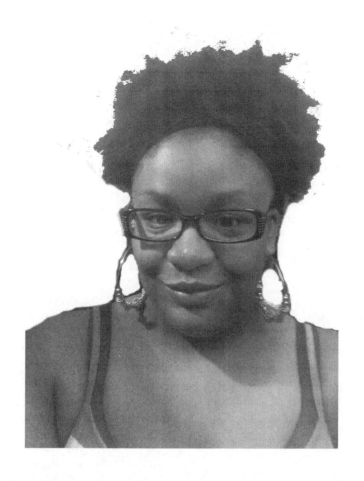

If you do small-medium twists your twists out will be curlier.

How To Do A Twists Out

After you've had your twists in for about 1-2 weeks, they'll start to look bad (strands of hair coming out of the twists). That's when you know it's time to take them out and do a twist out.

Step #1: Take out every single one of your twists.

Step #2: Style as desired.

You can use a headband. In the picture above I'm wearing a black satin scarf as a headband.

Headbands are really cute with twist outs.

But you can also wear your twists out without a headband, I've done that too.

Braid outs are also an option. Simply braid your hair the night before and follow the instructions above.

Fro

A fro is by far the easiest style you can do no matter how long your hair is. Fros look more tasteful if you put some type of headband on, but it depends on your hair type-- you may not need one.

I usually use scarves when I wear my fros. If you check out my <u>YouTube Channel</u> I show you a great way to do this, it's easy and it's definitely good for a lazy day.

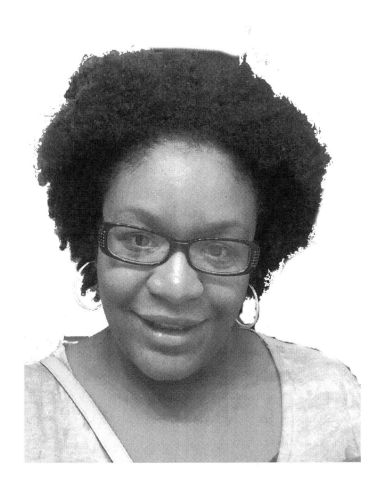

How To Do A Fro

Depending on the texture of your hair. All you
would have to do is wet your hair and it will curl up.

Then allow it to dry and put the scarf around it.

For shorter hair you can use a thin headband and just poof it out.

Step 1: Your hair can either be curly or kinky, just poof it out by taking different sections of your hair and pulling on them in an outward motion.

Step 2: Add a headband or scarf (optional).

Then that's basically it, you're good to go. For best results make sure your hair is oiled and not dry.

Braids

Braids are another popular and yet low maintenance style. You can have a lot of small mini braids, medium-sized, or even large ones.

The only braids I do myself are the ones where I do two braids going to the back.

Otherwise, I use weave in my hair when I get braids because the weave helps it to last longer. When it comes to doing a lot of braids, I don't have the skills, so I go to someone who does and pay them a few dollars.

**Side note: You can still wear weave and be

natural. I think of natural as not using relaxers or perms. Weaves are great for protective styles to help your hair grow.

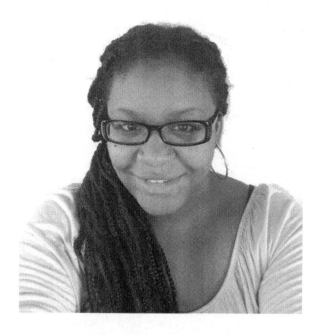

The Takeaway

Okay, so far we've gone over what products you need and how to style your hair. These are the two basic things you need to know how to do for a successful natural hair journey.

There are so many different types of styles you can do, but for beginners, I suggest sticking to the basics so you can make your hair healthy and grow it out.

Chapter 3: Keeping Your Hair Healthy

This is one of the most important chapters in the book. Healthy hair is what causes it to grow super long and begin to change the texture of your hair.

Deep Conditioning

Deep condition your hair anytime you're about to put in a new style. So if you're about to do your twists, deep condition your hair.

If you're about to wear it in a fro, make sure to deep condition. You cannot "over deep condition" your hair.

The more the better. Deep conditioning makes hair stronger, moisturizes it, and keeps it healthy, which in turn helps it to grow.

How To Deep Condition Your Hair

Materials You'll Need: Shower Cap, deep conditioner, conditioner, shampoo, leave in conditioner, access to water, towel, tea tree oil (optional), hair dryer (optional)

This process is pretty simple:

Step #1: Separate your hair into four even sections.

Step #2: Open your deep conditioner, take out a generous amount, and spread it all throughout one of your sections (make sure you get the roots and the ends).

Step #3: Add in any other hair softener, oils, moisturizers, or conditioners you want to that section; the more the better.

Step #4: Put conditioners in each of the other 3 sections.

Step #5: Add a small amount of tea tree oil to your scalp to prevent itching and increase moisture (optional). Put on a shower cap and let the conditioner sit on your hair for at least three hours.

To increase your results, you can sit under and drier or work out. Working out or putting your head under the dryer allows the pores in your scalp to open, and your hair to become more soft and manageable because of the heat.

Step #6: Rinse the conditioner out with a natural sulfate-free shampoo. Dry your hair with a microfiber towel or t-shirt and then you can add in some leave in conditioner.

After that, you're pretty much finished. A tip is to wash your hair out while it's still in sections so you can manage it better.

Deep conditioning makes your hair softer and untangles it.

Trimming Your Ends

To keep your hair healthy, you're going to have to keep your ends clipped. This allows for growth.

How To Trim Your Ends

Materials You'll Need: sharp scissors, wide toothed comb, ponytail holders, spray bottle, access to water

Step #1: Take a little manageable section out and

put the rest of your hair into a ponytail, clip, or out of the way.

Step #2: Fill your spray bottle with water. Take the strand you just separated and spray it with the water.

Step #3: Comb the strand thoroughly.

Step #4: Put the strand between two of your fingers so it's straight. Chop off the end of your hair that's not even.

That's pretty much the process. You want to play it by ear. I recommend trimming your ends every two months.

You don't have to pay someone to do this, you can do it yourself.

Hot Oil Treatment

Hot oil treatments are not something you have to do that often. I recommend doing these when you find your hair and scalp getting dry.

This is a more advanced process and takes a little more time, but it's worth it.

How To Do A Hot Oil Treatment

Materials you'll need: virgin olive oil, tea tree oil, a microwave, peppermint oil, spray bottle, access to water and sink, deep conditioner, squeeze bottle, bobby pins, dryer

Step 1: Take your spray bottle and fill it with water and wet your hair thoroughly.

Step 2: Separate your hair into six even sections (3 on each side).

Step 3: Take one section out and take your spray bottle and spray it very well. Then use your deep conditioner and run it through that section.

Step 4: Use your squeeze bottle and fill it almost to the top with the olive oil. Then add in a very small amount of tea tree oil and peppermint oil.

Take the squeeze bottle and squirt it on your scalp in the section you're working on. Rub the oil into your scalp. Then take some of the oil from the squeeze bottle and rub it through all the hair in that section.

Step 5: Twist the section you just finished and continue with all the other five sections with the same process.

Step 6: Take a bobby pin and take one of your

twists and pin it to the middle of your head. Repeat this for all the twists.

Step 7: Sit under the dryer for 30 minutes.

Step 8: Leave your hair in the twists and rinse out the oil treatment. Do this by placing your head in the sink and letting the water run over it.

Step 8: Shampoo your scalp as the water rinses over it. Add more conditioner and rinse out.

Then after that, you're pretty much finished.

Take Away

Make sure you're deep conditioning your hair every time you switch to a new style, or at least once a month.

Keep your ends clipped. Do this, at least, every two months or when you see that your ends are uneven.

When you find your hair or scalp getting dry, do a hot oil treatment.

Also, look into adding some essential oils to keep your hair moisturized:

- argan

- jojoba

- coconut

- olive

- flaxseed

Chapter 4: How To Grow Your Hair Long

Growing your hair long is a process, but it's definitely doable. There are many success stories of women whose hair went from short to long in just a matter of months.

You can grow your hair long by deciding right now that you want long hair and you'll do what it takes to take care of it and manage it well. So once you make that commitment to yourself, keep it.

There are many formulas and products out there that will allow your hair to grow, but if you just take care of it the right way-- it'll grow on its own.

To prevent breakage don't put any direct heat to your hair. This means no flat ironing or hot combing. There is a safe way to do this, so if you are going to blow out your hair I suggest going to a professional that knows about natural hair growth.

Never put a relaxer in your hair. Relaxers will destroy your hair if you don't take care of them. And a lot of times you can have a relaxer go wrong and a lot of your hair will fall out.

Not taking care of relaxed hair can cause your hair to dry out, and it can cause a lot of breakage.

Just stay clear of any relaxer or perm for that

matter. Especially if you want to go natural.

Use natural products and products that are sulfate free.

Keep up with your deep conditions, hot oil treatments, and keep your ends clipped.

Growing your hair is all about maintenance and keeping it healthy.

Don't neglect it, and you'll find that it'll be growing in no time.

"If you love it; it'll grow."

Check out Natural Hair Growth Secrets for more

tips on how to grow natural hair long:

http://www.amazon.com/Natural-Hair-Growth-Secrets-natural-ebook/dp/B00NJYNCQI/

Chapter 5: Maintaining Your Hair

Creating a routine and schedule for your hair is your best bet for growth and healthy hair.

Start planning in your calendar when you want to get your hair done and when you want to take it out. Also, schedule your hot oil treatments, deep conditions, and trimmings.

Stay true to your natural hair and keep away from relaxers and direct heat.

Deep condition your hair before styling it.

Do hot oil treatments when your scalp gets dry and itchy or your hair is starting to dry out.

Trim your hair every two months or when you see it starting to have some breakage or uneven ends.

Don't try to do too much when you're just starting out. You just need to know the basics, then you can venture into more complex hair styles.

But right now you should be focusing on growing and maintaining what you have.

This is a pretty simple process once you get it down packed.

Make sure to <u>watch videos</u> on how to do twists and make sure that you're not neglecting your hair.

When you have a protective style in, and it's not the time to take it out but you feel your hair is drying out, make sure to have some olive oil spray on hand that you can use to moisturize your hair.

You can also add plain water into a spray bottle and spray your hair daily. Your hair needs water just like your body needs water.

You can add essential oils and other moisturizers to a spray and make your own recipes. Keeping your hair moisturized will help it to grow and remain healthy.

If your scalp is drying out or itching while wearing a protective style; just add a small amount of tea tree oil or apple cider vinegar and that should take care of the problem.

Make sure to wrap your hair up at night using a silk or satin bonnet or pillow case.

Make taking care of your hair a habit, as long as you're not lazy about it and don't neglect your hair you should begin to see the results you want.

Conclusion

Thank you again for reading *The Beginners Guide To Natural Hair*. And congratulations on starting your natural hair journey!

I hope this book was able to help you to begin your natural hair journey successfully.

The next step is to buy some products and get started trying some natural hair styles.

hank You!

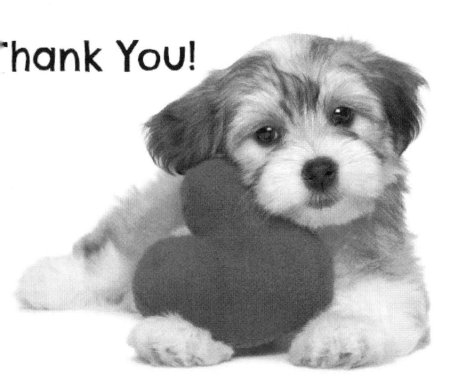

Finally, if you enjoyed this book, then I'd like to ask you for a favor, would you be kind enough to leave a review for this book on Amazon? It'd be greatly appreciated!

Your review will give me feedback on the book, tips on how to improve it or a pat on the back for a job well done. Plus, it helps other naturals find the book. Thank you and good luck!

Preview Of 'Natural Hair Growth Secrets'

Chapter 1: How To Care For Natural Hair

The best way to grow your hair is to take very good care of it. If you procrastinate and don't take the proper care, your hair will not grow any longer.

We all get lazy at times. Sometimes when it's time to do my twists over, I simply don't feel like it. But when it comes down to it, **you will get out of it what you put into it.**

If you use the methods in this book, your hair will grow, and it will grow consistently long. It's up to you to apply what you learn.

Treatments

To grow your hair, you will need to treat it. How often will vary depending on your hair style. But ultimately you should be treating your hair every 2 weeks.

When I say treatments I mean pre-pooing, shampooing, washing, conditioning, hot oil treatments, and trimming.

Pre-Poo

A pre-poo is what you do before shampooing your hair. This prepares your hair for the shampooing which can be very harsh and strip your hair.

A pre-poo is optional, but I recommend you do it because it makes your hair much easier to untangle.

What you will need: a moisturizing conditioner, natural oils such as extra virgin olive oil or coconut oil, shower cap or plastic shopping bag

A pre-poo is pretty similar to a deep condition but less complicated. The purpose of the pre-poo is to prepare your hair to be washed.

Step 1: Separate your hair into manageable sections (4-8 depending on length). Do this by sectioning off your hair into ponytails, knots, or twists.

Step 2: Take out one section of your hair that you want to work on first. Grab your conditioner or natural oils or a mixture of both and apply it to the section. Once the section is finished put it back into a ponytail.

Step 3: Apply the oils and conditioner generously to the section by either spraying or rubbing it into your hair. If applying directly from the bottle into your hands-- make sure you're making a root to tip motion.

Step 4: Repeat the process with all sections of your head.

Step 5: Put on a shower cap or plastic shopping bag to enclose the conditioner and oils. Let sit for 45min-2hours.

Step 6: Take your hair out of the shower cap or plastic bag and, while it's still in its sections, rinse it out using cold water. This will seal in the moisture and close the cuticles.

Step 7: Go on to your shampoo routine.

Click here to check out the rest of Natural Hair Growth Secrets on Amazon

Or go to www.naturalhairmaster.com/resources/

Check Out My Other Books

Below you'll find some of my other popular natural hair books that are popular on Amazon and Kindle as well. Simply click on the links below to check them out. Alternatively, you can visit my author page on Amazon to see other work done by me.

<u>Natural Hair Growth Secrets: How To Grow Natural Hair Long</u>

<u>Natural Hair Recipes: Do It Yourself Natural Hair Products</u>

<u>Natural Hair Transitioning: The Complete Guide To Transitioning From Relaxed To Natural Hair</u>

<u>The Big Chop: Guide To Starting Your Natural Hair Journey From Scratch</u>

If the links do not work, for whatever reason, you can simply search for these titles on the Amazon website to find them. Visit http://www.naturalhairmaster.com/resources/ for more books and guides on natural hair.

Natural Hair Checklist & Journal [FREE]

Our printable checklist provides you with a list of everything you'll need to begin your natural hair journey.

Take it with you on the go, it can be downloaded on any device.

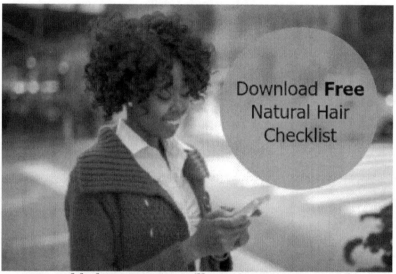

Download **Free** Natural Hair Checklist

As an added **BONUS** you'll receive our **Natural Hair Journey Journal**. A digital journal where you can track your experiences of growth, recipes, and more.

To Download Visit:
www.naturalhairmaster.com/naturalhaircheckli standjournal

About The Author

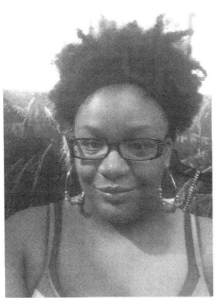

Hello, my name is Argena Hall and I'm here because I am passionate about helping women on their natural hair journey.

I know what it is like to be confused about where to start and not knowing what products you need and how to style your own natural hair.

It wasn't long ago that I was searching online for natural hair tutorials and trying to figure out where to start.

Then I discovered a way to start going natural and doing my own hair.

It hasn't always been easy. I have run into problems like not knowing what twisting creams to use or if I should get the "big chop".

Now I've been natural for three whole years! And my hair has been growing like crazy.

And now I want to help you to get the same results. The first step is simple, download my free beginners natural hair checklist to ensure you purchase the right products to get started with your natural hair journey.

Made in the USA
Middletown, DE
18 June 2016